Don't Inflict Emotional Torture

Change your Eating Habits
And Live a Healthy Lifestyle

By: Sue Feldman (Nutritionist)

Medical Disclaimer
       Page: 3
Introduction – My story
       Page: 5
Chapter 1 - Changing Your Eating Habits
       Page: 8
Chapter 2 - A Look Back
       Page: 16
Chapter 3 - In Everyday Life
       Page: 19
Chapter 4 - Rules to Consider
       Page: 24
Chapter 5 - The Easiest Way to Change
       Page: 28
Chapter 6 - Changing For Free
       Page: 31
Chapter 7 - Changing - Step by Step
       Page: 35
Chapter 8 - Strategies to Changing
       Page: 39
Chapter 9 - Tips to Change Successfully
       Page: 44
Chapter 10 - Common Questions Changing
       Page: 49
Chapter 11 – 4 Eating Plans
       Page: 54
Chapter 12 – The Food Lists
       Page: 60

Medical Disclaimer:

The information in this book is not intended to replace a 1-on-1 relationship with a qualified medical professional and it is not intended as medical advice. It is intended as a sharing of knowledge and information. I encourage you to make your own health core decisions based upon your research and in partnership with your doctor. You know your body and how it feels; sometimes a sore in your side might be more than a pulled muscle. So taking a pain killer tablet might help the pain but not cure the underlining reason why you got the pain in the first place. Self-diagnose, is the first step, know thy self. You can become a healthier, happier and more successful person by making a few simple changes to your lifestyle, and eating habits.

This publication is part of a series of products and publications.

Introduction – My story

I have been a Nutritionist since 1998 and been interested in health issues all my life. I believe that we need to take extra vitamins and minerals supplements, as the fresh food we eat today is not as healthy as in our grand parents' days; our soil has been depleted of minerals from mass production.

I have to say this: that it's your body and if something does not feel right get to the bottom of it - go for blood tests or even x-rays to get answers. General Practitioners, GP's, only study about 3 to 5% of nutrition in all the years they study to become doctors. You can become a healthier, happier and more successful person by making a few simple changes to your eating habits and lifestyle.

Don't be the person who misses out on the opportunities in life because you don't understand the necessary principles of healthy living. Be the kind of person others marvel at. Be the kind of person other people see and say "I don't know how you stay and look so good". Be the kind of person who takes action.

The information in this book is intended as a sharing of knowledge and information. I encourage you to make your own health core decisions.

My health has been a consistent feature in my life. Since I was a kid, what I remember, is that my father was ill for most of my childhood. I used to nurse him and help whenever I could. He was in and out of hospital, so I never knew if he would be home when I got back from school. To cut a long story short, he suffered from diabetics, heart problems (9 coronaries) and high cholesterol, ate lots of very rich and unhealthy foods, and smoked like a trouper.

He ended up getting gangrene on this toes and had to have his legs, from his knees down, amputated. At the time of the first operation, the surgeon started on his better leg, but my dad had a heart attack on the operation table, so they did not amputate both legs.

They had to stop and send him home with only completing half of the removal. He lived another 4 years with his bad leg then went for the second operation and died on the table. I was 11 years old!

I also had a sister who lives with a weight problem and since she was 6 months old she was put on diet. I vowed as a kid that I would never be fat, and I have lived my whole life making sure mentally and physically that I would be slim and trim. My whole family is on the larger size of their idea weight, but not me.

So I decided to study as much as possible about Health. Then in 1998 I completed a course in a creditable manner and furnished satisfactory evidence of proficiency in Nutritional Therapy and have been entered upon the Register of the Complementary Health Studies Centre.

Hence writing this book to share what I know with others, so that they can become better and healthier and live a happy lifestyle.

Chapter 1

Changing Your Eating Habits

This is not about going on a 'diet' to lose a few kilos or pounds, which I am sure you have tried in the past. You decide on a diet plan, stick with it for a couple of weeks or a month, and maybe get to your goal weight. Then you go back to your 'normal eating habits'. So what happens then – wham, bang, and crash you are back to where you were before, or even bigger! Many have called this 'The Yo-Yo diet'!

Therefore don't go on a Diet – change your mind-set and eating habits!

Think of the word 'Diet' as:

Don't inflict emotional torture on your body and mind trying to get it healthy, as soon as you think or someone says you need to go on a 'diet' your mind rebels and all of a sudden you are craving (a killer crave like an addiction) for everything that you are *not supposed* to eat. Therefore *don't die for it*. Simply change to a healthy eating plan. Notice what you eat because 'you *are* what you eat'.

Remember this: - "If you always do what you always did, you'll always get what you always got".

Typically when a person thinks of changing their eating habits, they reflect on being obsessive with food. The reality is that the two could be completely opposite. Provided you are trying to live a healthy lifestyle, there are a few measures you must make in order to reach your objectives.

Today the biggest problem is that 'fat' has been taken out of some foods, but to preserve it the companies had to add 'sugar'. Sugar is poison to your body – it destroys your teeth, it makes you fat, and it causes untold diseases and disease.
Sugar does not give you energy in the long run, its gives you a false high, then when it is burnt off you need another fix (of sugar). Sugar is really an addiction - so if you need energy have protein instead, as it is the fuel for your body.

Your life should be run like a fancy car – when people pay for an expensive car they look after it. It is done by putting in the right gas or petrol, clean water and good oil. One does not buy a car to stand in the garage just to look pretty; it needs to be driven (exercised). And of course it is kept clean and the outside is waxed to keep it shiny, like new.

So why do we not look after our body like that? The body needs the right gas (called proteins), clean water and good oil or fats. And our body needs to be cleansed (a Detox program, see chapter 11) and the wax is doing exercises or just being active.

Following are some tips to push you to begin:

-- *Thinking and seeing yourself as slim and healthy*

If you change the way you look at things, the things you look at change.

DR. WAYNE DYER

WWW.VERYBESTQUOTES.COM

The biggest mistake, which anyone could experience when attempting to change their eating habit, is falling short with this vital tip. If you choose to not observe yourself as slim and healthy, it will be difficult. That is how dependent it is to changing your eating habit is on thinking and seeing yourself as slim and healthy.

In case you are curious how to think and see yourself as slim and healthy, then don't weigh yourself on a daily basis. If you are overweight use a pair of jeans or a belt to measure if you have lost any weight along the way of eating the right kind of healthy foods. Love yourself and think yourself slim!

Power of using your mind! Use energy to focus on your ideal body, remember if you focus on the negative that's what you will get, so see and believe what you want and eventually you will get it. The ideal body for you!

-- Making choices that are right for you and not conforming to others

Making choices isn't always easy. But, you always have a choice.

[www.christieinge.com]

Making choices that are right for you and not conforming to others helps you change your eating habits. Understandably, it could be hard to get in the habit of doing it. Begin by making choices that are right and not conforming to what is just dished up every day, and it ought to become force of habit when you change your eating habits.

-- Having healthy eating options

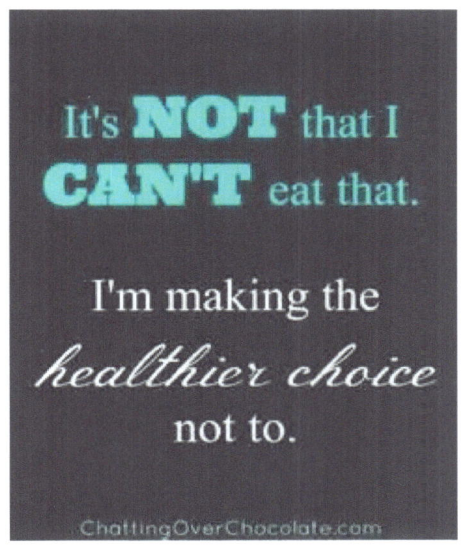

An integral part of the foundation that is necessary to change your eating habits involves having healthy eating options. When you have healthy eating option, it allows you to be in an appropriate mind-set to achieve the utmost goal of changing.

Although we will help you prepare looking at what you eat differently, you initially need to make sure that changing your eating habits is appropriate for you. Looking at what you eat differently is the key, and you must think about it before going forward.

Since you recognize that you are in the right mind-set to change your eating habits, we can examine certain preliminary practices that one would already be doing. Use that opportunity to draw in these practices into your life because it will make preparing to change easier.

One of the best ways to determine whether you will be capable to change is to analyze the day-to-day practices of folks who have already changed their eating habits. You would not need to emulate their accomplishments all at once, as that would be difficult.

Yet, you must be equipped to put forth as much time as they do. Imitate their practices, as they are exactly where you want to be. In addition, reflect on these questions:

Are your eating habits the same as your family (do you all have the same health/weight problems)?

Are you addicted to junk food? (Are all your meals take-outs?)

Is your body slowing down with aches and pain?

Ideally, you replied positively to these questions. Then probably changing your eating habits is an appropriate activity for you. Congratulations for committing to that initial step forward toward accomplishing your goals by continuing to read!

Changing your eating habits takes heaps of effort invested over time. As you can see, the best way to get equipped for changing your eating habits is to offer yourself the suggested timeframe for your footwork so you can prevail. Do that, and changing your eating habits could be much easier.

Chapter 2

Changing Your Eating Habits - A Look Back

Realize that you aren't the first person in the world that has the goal of changing your eating habits. In fact, there are tons of men and women all over that want to look at what they eat differently. The indisputable reality is that only a handful of people will really make the commitment and accomplish it.

Usually people, who do change, do so because of a health issue, like having cancer, or getting diabetes or a heart attack. Changing sooner rather than later before dis-eases set-in is a good idea.

Don't think of being obsessive with food. Eat 3 meals a day, to keep yourself energized. Drink plenty of water when you feel hungry, as water can give you a feeling of being full. Changing your eating habits necessitates one to be changeable and steadfast. We recognize this.

Now we are prepared to analyze the stages recommended with changing your eating habits so we can enjoy our future accomplishments.
If you study others who have done well in changing their eating habits either now or long ago, you will discover one thing in common among the personalities who have done well.

They knew what was recommended before starting, and they appreciated what type of person is likely to prevail. When you recognize what kind of individual is necessary to change, determined and committed, there is not anyone that will block the path between you and your success!

Being entirely focused to change your eating habits requires dedication mentally, along with physically. The number one method to train all around is to have a strong mentality and get mentally prepared.

You should probably take this time to check whether you have the gumption it takes. Do you have a changeable personality? It is a vital part of the formula that everyone who expects to change their eating habits needs, or else looking at what you eat differently will get ridiculously hard, if not unfeasible.

Additionally make sure you have the drive that changing your eating habits will take. Are your eating habits the same as your family (do you all have the same health/weight problems)? There could be a major difference between contemplating something as a beneficial idea and ultimately doing it. Without a doubt, you'd need a ton of discipline, desire, willpower and determination to move forward.

You've already taken a big step towards being equipped to change your eating habits. Some people botch up for good reason. They simply did not recognize what precisely they were getting themselves into.

Changing your eating habits is that one thing in life that necessitates you to get entirely steadfast and prepared. Through looking forward and making sure you are changeable and beneficial, you would be taking the first step toward preparing.

Also consider that choosing to change is equally important to your health success. Your mind might try to persuade you that changing your eating habits could be rather hard or is probably not worth the effort, but by choosing to change and maintaining concentration on your goal, you will do it! Let's determine how we will now plan for changing your eating habits!

Chapter 3

Changing Your Eating Habits in Everyday Life

During the time you look at what you eat for 1 week, by writing down every morsel that passes your lips, you would discover that changing your eating habits is impacting other aspects of your life. Changing your eating habits is a major lifestyle choice that impacts you in many ways.
If you can think back to when we initially started the progression of changing your eating habits, you probably remember being presented with three questions:

Are your eating habits the same as your family (do you all have the same health/weight problems)?

Are you addicted to junk food? (Are all your meals take-outs?)

Is your body slowing down with aches and pain?

Along with looking at your lifestyle, these questions are also looking to analyze your skills and desires. So if you replied yes to these questions, there is an indication of what is significant to you.

By noting the role these qualities play in your daily life, you are acknowledging the role that changing your eating habits plays in life. Changing what you are eating now is not easy. All rewarding activities necessitate commitment. Changing your eating habits is no exception.

One of the hardest ways to change is if you are a person who enjoys baking. Look at the kind of food you are making, do you use a load of sugar and keep tasting as you are preparing? There are many recipes on the market that do not use sugar, and they are usually diabetic recipes and very delicious too. Most people cannot tell the difference.

Be sure to look at what is necessary before changing. This is exactly what will be impacting in other areas of your life. Making choices that are right for you and not conforming to others, having healthy eating options and thinking and seeing yourself as slim and healthy ought to be seen as acts that overlap looking at what you eat differently. Even though we would be examining this as being specific to changing your eating habits, much of it will change other areas in your life.

The best thing about changing your eating habits is the changeable characteristic that is necessary to succeed which will make its way in all aspects of life. That prepares you to become a more changeable person overall. Anytime you look at what you eat differently, adding some exercise and thinking of your feelings you would be preparing your spirit for what will follow. It is just one of the good things of changing.

One may have a beneficial characteristic to change too. That is one more attribute which impacts your lifestyle. The longer you call on that attribute to look at what you eat differently, the more you will recognize that attribute within unrelated areas of your life.

Changing your eating habits really takes much more out of one than one may think. Changing your eating habits is not only something to try; it is alternatively an entire lifestyle shift. It clearly takes a distinctive set of qualities to change your eating habits successfully and sticking with it.

If you are devoted to completing whatever you begin, having the willpower, changing your eating habits will become another amazing thing which you accomplish in your life. Congratulations with beginning your progression towards a more satisfying healthy lifestyle! Read chapter 11 to give you some ideas on different plans which you could try for yourself.

Chapter 4

Rules to Consider While Changing Your Eating Habits

As we've recently analyzed, changing your eating habits requires quite a bit out of an individual. You should become changeable, beneficial, and determined. Some people may have these traits, but the reality is that preparing for a journey as impacting as changing your eating habits may really strip these traits away from you. Following are a handful of tips you ought to follow that will help your mind nurture these traits.

Preparing yourself for the difficult task of changing your eating habits is time-consuming and you will probably be putting in close to a couple of weeks to prepare. This ought to offer you enough time to ingrain these tips in your regiment.

Just remember 'you are what you eat' so cut out sugar and drink lots of water, this will keep your body hydrated and refreshed. It is one of the outcomes that this guideline will generate. Additionally, you will know what you need to do for you, particularly when the time arrives to actually forming new eating habits on a regular basis.

Also, remember that people who productively know what is 'healthy' will generally keep a journal or food diary and celebrate milestones. So to help you: order your Colouring Journal and Food Diary on Amazon. It is astonishing how these straightforward guidelines can be such a vital part in a larger goal.

When you see yourself as one who is beneficial, then you may find it relatively simple to incorporate these tips into your regimented process. Additionally, if you choose to keep a journal or food diary and celebrate milestones, then it will foster a feeling of accomplishment as you reach your goals.

Let us not forget our goal of being determined to improve your lifestyle and health. It could need yet another degree of energy during the preparation stage, but it'll be worth it. During the time you are working toward getting into smart routines and getting into good eating habits and drinking water often, you should probably remain with a positive attitude and outlook to living a healthy lifestyle.

Through ascertaining that you maintain this mind-set and willpower, you should dissuade your mind from becoming discouraged and giving up.

Changing how you eat is not being obsessive with food. Even though any person can try to look at what you eat differently, it requires one who's determined and changeable to ultimately accomplish this goal of changing your eating habits.

When making a vow to thoroughly prepare, it is your responsibility to not drop out! Do you remember when you were asked these specific questions?

Are your eating habits the same as your family (do you all have the same health/weight problems)?

Are you addicted to junk food? (Are all your meals take-outs?)

Is your body slowing down with aches and pain?

To each of those questions, you replied yes. This is excellent because we had to determine whether or not you were determined, changeable and motivated. It is these qualities that will steer you to your success when you finally change your eating habits. So, remember to choose to change, know what is healthy, and be determined to improve your lifestyle and health. Follow the above tips and you will be a healthy and happy person in no time!

Chapter 5

The Easiest Way to Change Your Eating Habits

There are many methods that folks use to change their eating habits. By now, you ought to know that preparation is vital to being successful. Say you are searching for the best method to change your eating habits, and then be sure to offer yourself ample time to find it. Once you do, schedule time to look at what you eat. Usually, 1 week is a standard period of time to accomplish that goal, by seeing what you are eating on a daily basis in your journal or food diary. Is it junk or healthy food?

You're now ultimately ready to get into the task at hand. However, first we will examine a few beneficial habits. That way you are as equipped as possible the moment you decide to change your eating habits.

The three steps that you ought to do to prepare to change are: make choices that are right for you and not conforming to others, have healthy eating options and think and see yourself as slim and healthy. Combined these tips make a strong core for your footwork.

Preparing for at least 1 week before you change your eating habits is absolutely important, and can't be overemphasized. It will show you how and what you are eating that is not healthy in your food journal or diary. It permits you to wholly prepare.

Additionally, it certainly gives you all of the beneficial practices necessary for changing. You would discover that choosing to change, knowing what is healthy, and being determined to improve your lifestyle and health will assure that you put forth your best effort possible.

When you disregard these actions, you will forego knowing what you need to do for you, knowing the benefits of healthy eating, and feeling fit and healthy all the time. These results all result from the preparation phase.

With the right scheduling and process, you will certainly be boosting energy, getting into smart routines along with getting into good eating habits and drinking water often. All of these are definitely important to do to change.

The best part of it is: if you can put forth a bit of time into preparing, then it should ultimately get quite simple for you. So keep from scurrying through any introductory phases. And conclusively, make sure that you are completely ready.

Many folks wrongfully think that it could be hard, or even impossible to become a healthy and vibrant person. Realistically, it just requires one who is changeable, has the willpower, beneficial and determined to ultimately go through the introductory steps.

If you can entirely commit to rejecting short-cuts in the preparation stage and perform all of the steps successfully, then you are better positioned to change your eating habits.

The best method to changing your eating habits is to reflect all of the steps laid out here. Consequentially, cutting corners is certainly not worth the time and must be avoided while looking at what you eat differently.

You must focus your effort on the first phase of the process as it would make you more productive. The reality is 1 week is actually not a large amount of time to prepare for such an impacting event as changing your eating habits. So, make the vow to change, put forth the expected amount of time, and you can be changing your eating habits in no time!

Chapter 6

Changing Your Eating Habits For Free

You may think that it costs a good deal of money to change your eating habits, but in fact you can look at what you eat differently for free. The thing you ought to do when you want to look at what you eat differently is to remove any existing thoughts you may have about what it is like.

Instead, concentrate your time on the groundwork. Also consider, choosing to change, knowing what is healthy, and being determined to improve your lifestyle and health can be integral ways to get equipped for changing your eating habits without necessarily having to go broke. Don't spend money on fancy diets or joining slimming clubs. 'Know thy self' and what you are putting into your mouth.

There are practical things you may also try, in order to squander little money. Invest in healthy recipe books or go on-line to find healthy eating plans, or follow one of the eating plans in chapter 11. It is not a diet you are looking for, but a good eating plan. You would not have to put forth a good deal of money to look at what you eat differently. This is a simple option when your objectives are the focal point.

During the time you are being determined to improve your lifestyle and health, do it with a mind-set to save money. Read about the ingredients on package foods. If there is a high sugar content - don't buy it.

During the time you are changing your eating habits you do not have to blow money on overly high-priced food items when there are economical alternatives which work just as effectively. Crowds of people had been changing their eating habits before many of the more high-priced food items were available. If they did not require it, then you would not either.

The best suggestion is to just keep your center of attention as the top priority. More exactly, choosing to change, knowing what is healthy along with being determined to improve your lifestyle and health are actions you should probably focus your attention. During the time you really analyze your feelings, it is increasingly easier to identify when you are addicted to junk food and on things you would not need to eat.

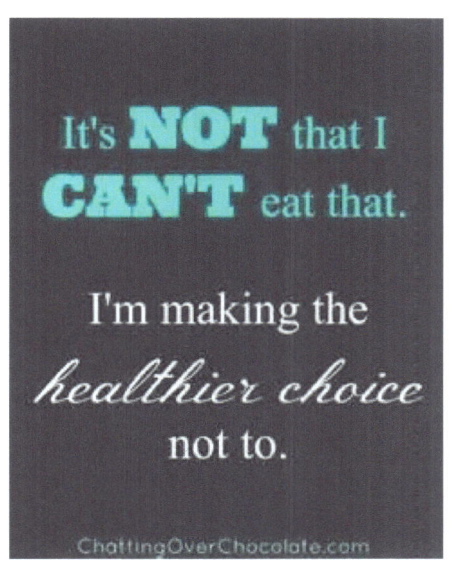

It's **NOT** that I **CAN'T** eat that.

I'm making the *healthier choice* not to.

ChattingOverChocolate.com

When you take the effort in preparing, you ought to know what you need to do *for you*, which is one of the key goals for changing your eating habits. Choosing to change does not necessitate spending a good deal cf money.

Choosing to change involves getting in the habit of knowing what a healthy way to eat is. And many times it may look extremely high-priced, but you can know what is healthy without going broke. Knowing what is healthy motivates you to know what food you are putting in your mouth. It can be accomplished very affordably.

Finally, concentrate a bit of time on knowing what is healthy, along with how you ought to be determined to improve your lifestyle and health properly. Do not allow yourself to get tempted by companies which require you to pay membership fees. Remember, there would be adequate alternatives available to be determined to improve your lifestyle and health that are nearly free in cost.

Nevertheless, you must generally determine where you would spend your money by thinking of your key goal of changing your eating habits. Your feelings will play a large role in regards to this. You may be hunting for an effective method to change your eating habits. Through recognizing this, you ought to make a good deal of progress toward your goal.

Chapter 7

Changing Your Eating Habits - Step by Step

At this point, it is understood which specific kind of person it takes to productively change their eating habits. We've also learned more about the qualities that one needs in order to look at what you can eat differently. So today, we can now get started with what exactly we are set to accomplish.

Without a doubt, the first step is verifying that you are definitely choosing to change as it can determine your readiness to change your eating habits. You ought to think of choosing to change just like this: no person can truthfully look at what they eat differently without choosing to change. It is literally impossible - that is just how essential this step is.

Choosing to change is also essential if you want to become productive. It will also result with you knowing what you need to do for you and knowing the benefits of healthy eating. The moment you start out choosing to change, you will have a ton to gain, health wise, and absolutely nothing to lose! (Or maybe lose a little extra weight).

You also need to continue knowing what is healthy throughout your preparations, and when to change your eating habits. To look at what you eat differently is undoubtedly hard, however knowing what is healthy ought to help. Plus, choosing to change will help you start boosting vitality, which is clearly important. Boosting vitality ought to help you when you look at what you eat differently now and in the days ahead.

Knowing what is healthy also provides more benefits in unique ways outside of changing your eating habits. It should help you know what food you are putting in your mouth and learn what others have gained by eating healthily.

Also knowing what food you are putting in your mouth is equally important whether you are changing your eating habits or not. So, you should probably consider implementing any method that results in you knowing what foods are the best to eat.

You may feel ready for changing your eating habits in less than a week once you begin choosing to change, particularly if you know what is healthy.

Typically, 1 week is the approximate period of time which people plan for getting ready to change by analyzing your food journal or diary to find your bad eating habits. Remember these averages when you are calculating your timelines.

Another aspect that is necessary to help you become successful with changing your eating habits is being determined to improve your lifestyle and health. You would not have to narrow in on being determined to improve your lifestyle and health until the second part of your preparations, though certainly do not move past it altogether.

Being determined to improve your lifestyle and health ought to assist you to boost energy, which could be beneficial for your preparations. It also encourages you to get into smart routines and get into good eating habits and drinking water often, which in turn encourages you to change your eating habits.

Finally, you'd be equipped to change your eating habits by choosing to change, knowing what is healthy and being determined to improve your lifestyle and health. It generally requires a week of planning getting truly ready. But, that period of time ought to go by really rapidly.

If you can schedule a fixed date to start your preparation period and mark 1 week later, then it'll lead your brain to see that timeframe as the introductory phase, like setting a goal. At that point, you will be prepared to narrow in on choosing to change, along with knowing what is healthy. Then, you will discover that your entire mind is truly ready to change your eating habits!

Chapter 8

Strategies to Changing Your Eating Habits

Changing your eating habits takes a ton out of an individual. Unfortunately, everyone does not really possess what it takes. There are some clear-cut methods that work more powerfully than others to assure that you are unfailingly preparing for your success the best way.

I tell people that you are not going on a 'diet' to change your eating habits, but starting a 'healthy eating plan'. Acknowledging this ought to lead you to finally change your eating habits.

Looking at what you eat differently needs one to become committed. One that is unchangeable, or has an addiction, might probably not become as successful as they could possibly be. These qualities are inside one who would have said no when approached with the question:

Are your eating habits the same as your family (do you all have the same health/weight problems)?

There are qualities for which anybody hoping to change their eating habits must have, and being changeable is one of them. The logic behind it is simple. Maintaining a changeable personality is exactly what empowers you to declare yourself as a healthy person after you productively change your eating habits.

Everyone can say that they want to change their eating habits. However, changing is a large step above being obsessive with food. One does not entail a good deal of preparation, and preparation is definitely important to the overall success with the other.

Looking at what you eat differently requires making choices that are right for you and not conforming to others. That may not seem like a big deal, when compared to changing your eating habits, but making choices that are right for you and not conforming to others is very important when you change your eating habits.

Having healthy eating options may be a no-brainer only because it is extremely vital for overall success when you change your eating habits. Having healthy eating options is important while you look at what you eat differently simply due to what is needed.

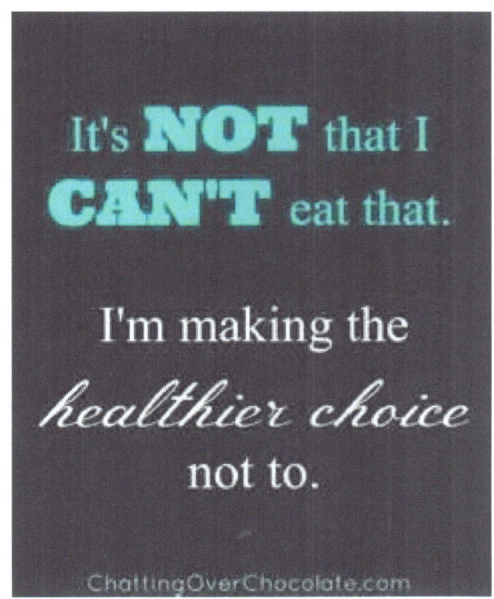

Thinking and seeing yourself as slim and healthy might also not seem like a big thing, however it certainly is. It is a mind-set, focus on what you want to achieve in the long term.

When changing your eating habits, you will need the footwork which you invested time on.
The methods to changing your eating habits help not only the goal of looking at what you eat differently, but each step really comes with a variety of benefits which will complement other aspects of your lifestyle.

It is simple to determine that knowing what you need to do for you is not only an advantage to changing your eating habits, but for life overall. Similarly, boosting vitality is well-known to help other areas of life.

Even boosting energy will become impacting outside of changing your eating habits. Other than being a lifestyle, some people will enjoy how changing their eating habits improves their lifestyle overall.

You might discover when you use these methods to change your eating habits that any existing qualities you had will become significantly enhanced.

Those who are changeable become even more changeable. Similarly, individuals who are beneficial seem even more beneficial. These are among the multiple specific reasons to get started changing your eating habits now!

Chapter 9

Tips to Change Your Eating Habits Successfully

Once you totally commit to changing your eating habits, there are many things that you can try to look at what you eat differently successfully. Here are a handful of tips which will help in changing your eating habits:

> ➤ Choosing to change has already been examined in great depth, and that is rather important when you are changing your eating habits. Make sure that you keep your body hydrated and refreshed. Additionally, make it a habit to remember 'you are what you eat' and drink lots of water. This does not only affect changing your eating habits, it actually affects your lifestyle in general.

> ➤ You should know that knowing what is healthy is important as well. It may get hard to make happen on your own. So a great method to foster a feeling of accomplishment as you reach your goals is to keep a journal or food diary and celebrate milestones. This ought to offer

you more drive to know what is healthy as you prepare to change your eating habits.

➢ Additionally, know that changing your eating habits needs you to constantly be determined to improve your lifestyle and health. In order to dissuade your mind from becoming discouraged and giving up, it is advisable to remain with a positive attitude and outlook to living a healthy lifestyle.

During the time you reflect these simple tips in your preparation of changing your eating habits, you will discover that you are gaining many benefits. Following are certain benefits which you may recognize as soon as you pursue your commitments to change your eating habits:

➢ Keep in mind knowing what you need to do for you will happen much more as long as you are choosing to change.

➢ Choosing to change equally permits your body to start knowing the benefits of healthy eating.

➢ Provided you know what is healthy, it ought to boost vitality.

➢ Additionally, knowing what is healthy helps with knowing what foods you are putting in your mouth.

➢ Through preparing to change your eating habits, and doing some exercise, you can be determined to improve your lifestyle and health and will boost energy because of it.

➢ Being determined to improve your lifestyle and health also will get you into smart routines, and setting goals.

Looking at what you eat differently certainly gives a ton of direct benefits, a handful of which we have examined, learning what others have gained by eating healthily, and feeling fit and healthy all the time, all occur when you are choosing to change, knowing what is healthy, and being determined to improve your lifestyle and health.

Looking at what you eat differently involves doing all of these things and basking in the benefits that follow. Additionally, following are a handful of additional tips:

> Don't spend money on fancy equipment. 'Know thy self' and what you are putting into your mouth.

> Invest in healthy recipe books or go on-line to find healthy eating plans or try the eating plans in chapter 11 of this book.

> Read about the ingredients in packaged food. If there is a high sugar content - don't buy it or eat it. Like sodas, chocolate, sweets, cakes and biscuits.

The moment you follow the advice included here, you'll be on track to look at what you can eat differently. Keep in mind to allow yourself a week to prepare. Having an adequate period of time to prepare is vital.

Part of the preparation is clearing out your food cupboards, get rid of the sweets, biscuits and the junk food, so you are not tempted to cheat, which will help your family as well.

What the eyes don't see, there is no temptation to have!

Any tips which would be noted here present a beginning point. The moment reviewing this information, you'll have an understanding of what it takes to change your eating habits. Feel free to add your individual observations and develop new instructions to push you to succeed.

Chapter 10

Common Questions about Changing Your Eating Habits

By now, you may be cognizant of the measures you must take to change your eating habits. Say you think of a question which hasn't been addressed, do not fret. Here are three common questions which surface with changing your eating habits:

Is it possible to change your eating habits for free?

For the most part, it is possible to change your eating habits for free. It is pointless to put forth heaps of money preparing to change. Following are a few tips to manage your budget.

> ➤ Don't spend money on fancy diet groups. 'Know thy self' and what you are putting into your mouth.

> ➤ Invest in healthy recipe bocks or go on-line to find healthy eating plans, or read what is healthy in chapter 11.

➤ Read about the ingredients on packaged food. If there is a high sugar content - don't buy it.

Another question which typically comes up when someone is planning to change your eating habits is about the common "rules" to consider while looking at what you eat differently. Following would be certain guidelines to bear in mind:

➤ While choosing to change, remember 'you are what you eat' and drink lots of water. This will keep your body hydrated and refreshed.

➤ Typically, knowing what is healthy is important when looking at what you eat. This will foster a feeling of accomplishment as you reach your goals.

➤ While you narrow in on being determined to improve your lifestyle and health, be sure to remain with a positive attitude, a strong willpower and outlook to living a healthy lifestyle. This will dissuade your mind from becoming discouraged and giving up.

You have taken the initial step toward changing your eating habits by reading more on it. Most likely additional questions may surface and one more way you may benefit yourself is by approaching this goal with a friend or family member that might have similar objectives.

At times a "buddy system" is a great solution while approaching a goal which requires a changeable and beneficial personality. Even though you could ultimately change your eating habits independently, it is advisable to connect with someone on a parallel progression to discuss questions as they surface, like family or friends.

Be mindful to pick like-minded companions and avoid people who may be addictive or unchangeable, as they would drive you away approaching your objectives.

Remember the questions you were asked just a bit ago?

Are your eating habits the same as your family (do you all have the same health/weight problems)?

Are you addicted to junk food? (Are all your meals take-outs?)

Is your body slowing down with aches and pain?

You have replied yes to the questions which determined you have the most effective personality to succeed at changing your eating habits. Choose a friend or family member that might also answer yes to these questions as they may also be inclined to succeed at changing their eating habits.

Chapter 11

4 Eating Plans

THE START OF CHANGING YOUR EATING HABITS:-

> Drink a cup of hot water and lemon/ginger juice first thing every morning.
> During the day drink 1,7 litres of water.
> Take multivitamin supplements every day, including (fresh – is best – swallow a small glove of garlic - like a tablet with liquids) or odourless garlic and see suggested list below.

__Juice Fast__: - Decide on the length (no longer than two or three days) of the fast and take only salads, juices and filtered or distilled Water for two days prior to the fast.

On the morning of the fast, start with a cup of boiling water and lemon juice, then take a glass of either freshly squeezed fruit or vegetable juice mixed 50/50 with water and sip it slowly.
For the duration of the day, have a glass of juice every two hours. You may alternate between fruit and vegetable juices, from the lists below, if you wish, but don't mix the two together.

General Fast: - For one week every two months, to help 'detox' your system, only eat food from the foods listed.

The Raw Food Eating Plan: - it is very simple and gives you lots of energy. As it states absolutely nothing is heated or cooked, you only eat food that is raw and natural.

It is fruit, vegetables and nuts. And you only eat when you feel hungry. Eat mixed salads either cut up or grated (even raw potatoes and beetroot).

Carry a bag of mixed nuts to snack on. When you go out with friends to a restaurant, you can feast from the salad bar (if they have one) or order a large salad as your main course. Most places now supply Smoothies so order one to your liking.

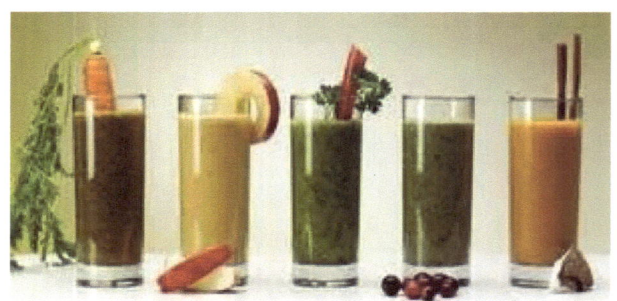

Healthy Eating: - To change your eating habits use the Food Lists to spice up what you eat instead. Thinking of the following tips:

> ➢ Remember that *breakfast* is the most important meal of the day, whether you have it first thing in the morning or at 10 a.m. or when you are ready, then lunch 4 or 5 hours later and then dinner 4 or 5 hours later. Meals to be spread out. A snack, twice a day but only if you feel hungry, it is not important to have if you don't feel like it.

> ➢ Drink plenty water and herbal teas throughout the day.

> ➢ Cut out all visible SUGARS (sweets, biscuits, cake, sugar in tea and coffee, use sweeteners instead, if you have to)

> ➢ Avoid fried foods and pastry in all forms but lightly stir-fried in olive oil is allowed.

> ➢ For fillers or snacks - Vegetables may be eaten freely, except avocado pears, baked/broad kidney and butter beans.

Fruits like grapefruit, lemons, limes, gooseberries, blackberries, raspberries and rhubarb (no sugar added) can be eaten freely. All other fruits 1 or 2 per day.

➢ *Miscellaneous foods* not on the list can be added. Clear soups, meat and yeast extracts, tomato juice, soda water, diet cold drinks and all herbs and spices, but not table salt.

➢ Now for the Naughty List – yes it is difficult to suddenly stop and change how you eat, so have <u>any TWO of these items twice a week</u>: - 1 glass of wine or 2 glasses low alcohol wine, 1 can (350ml) beer or 2 cans Lite beer, 1 tot measure spirits, 1 glass of sherry, 3 toffees, 1 scoop ice-cream or 2 scoops frozen yoghurt or sherbet ice-cream, 1 (150g) small bag of crisps, 1digestive biscuits 1 small Kit-Kat chocolate, (two fingers) but try to cut out chocolate all together.

➢ The <u>FOODS NOT ALLOWED LIST</u> below is for when you need to detox and improve your health. So, the items can be eaten in moderation, no more than once a day of each food listed *except* the Sugar – that needs to be cut out all together from your eating plan.

➤ There is not a *Meat List* because one should not eat meat when trying to get healthy. But if you do enjoy eating meats, do so only 2 or 3 times a week, but do not eat the fat, cut it off before cooking. Chicken or fish is a healthier alternate.

Chapter 12

THE FOOD LISTS

Foods that will increase the body's ability to heal yourself, improve your health and cleanse it (help with detoxing). Please remember don't eat anything that is not on these lists:

THE FRUIT LIST

Apples   Apricots   Blackberries
Blackcurrants   Blueberries   Cherries
Cranberries   Currants   Dates   Figs
Grapefruit   Grapes   Gooseberries
Greengages   Guavas   Kiwi fruit   Lemons
Limes   Loganberries   Lychees   Mangos
Melons   Mulberries   Nectarines
Passionfruit   Paw-paw   Pears   Pineapple
Pomegranates   plums   Prunes   Quinces
Raisins   Raspberries   Redcurrants
Rhubarb   Sultanas   Strawberries

THE VEGETABLE LIST

Vegetables to be eaten raw steamed or stir-fried in pure olive oil.

Artichokes   Asparagus   Aubergines
Beans (not lentils)   Beetroot   Bean Sprouts
Broccoli   Brussel sprouts   Cabbage
Carrots   Cauliflower   Celery   Chicory
Courgettes   Cucumber   Fennel   Kohlrabi
Leeks   Lettuce (all types)   Marrow
Onions   Parsnips   Peas   Peppers
Potatoes   Pumpkin   Radishes   Spring
Onions   Sweetcorn   Sweet potatoes
Squashes   turnips   Watercress   Yams.

NUTS LIST

Best eaten raw and unsalted.

Almonds   Brazils   Cashews   Chestnuts
Hazelnuts   Macadamia   Pecans   Pine
nuts   Pistachio   Walnuts   'Not allowed
Peanuts'

PULSE, SEED, HERB AND SPICE LIST

Alfalfa   Basil   Cardamom pods   Cayenne
pepper   Chick peas   Chilies   Chives
Coriander   Dill   Fennel   Ginger   Lemon
grass   Marjoram   Mint   Oregano
Parsley   Pepper – ground   Pumpkin seeds
Rosemary   Sage   Sesame   seeds
Sunflower seeds   Tarragon   Thyme

THE FISH LIST

Where possible eat fresh, or canned in olive/vegetable oil.

Cod   Crab   Haddock   Herring   Lemon
Sole   Lobster   Mackerel   Monkfish
Pilchards   Prawns   Salmon   Sardines
Scampi   Shrimps   Skate   Trout   Tuna

DRINKS LIST

Herbal teas (any)   Lemon/Ginger   Water

MISCELLANEOUS FOODS

Brown rice (short grain)   Balsamic vinegar
Cider vinegar   Grapeseed oil   Mustard grain
Olive oil   Olives (any)   Rice cakes –
unsalted and no sugar   Seaweed   Sesame
oil   Tofu   Walnut oil   Hummus

Suggested VITAMINS LIST

Please understand that you will not feel the benefits of supplements taking them for a week or so, it is a long term regiment to keep up. For every year that you have <u>not</u> taken supplements in your life time, it will take a month per each year to catch up and feel the true benefits of taking daily supplements.

- ✓ Chromium picolinate – reduces sugar cravings by stabilizing the metabolism of simple carbohydrates (sugar). 1 daily in the a.m.

- ✓ Lecithin capsules – is a fat emulsifier; breaks down fat so it can be removed from your body. 1 at each meal.

- ✓ Spirulina – excellent source of usable protein. Contains needed nutrients and stabilizes blood sugar. 1 between each meal.

- ✓ Vitamin C – a minimum of 1000 mg daily. It is necessary for normal glandular function. It speeds up a slow metabolism, prompting it to burn more calories and good for your immune system. 3 times per day.

- ✓ Vitamin B complex – It is need for proper digestion and gives you energy. 3 times per day.

- ✓ Kelp tablets - is a rich source the B vitamins, minerals and trace elements. (Do not take if you are allergic to iodine). 3 daily.

- ✓ Zinc – not more than 80 mg daily. It enhances the effectiveness of insulin and boosts the immune function. 1 before meals.

Please always remember to read the instruction given with each vitamin. If it states that the dose is the recommended daily allowance RDA – I recommend you take the RDA given and add a couple extra per day to get the full benefit.

FOODS NOT ALLOWED

Avocados, Bananas, Peanuts = Too much starch and fat

Bread, Rolls = Gluten in wheat flour difficult to digest

Caffeine = Chemical stimulant

Chocolate, Sweets = Too much sugar and fats

Cow's Milk/Cheese etc. = Lactose (milk sugars) difficult to digest

Lentils = Too much gas

Mushrooms = Too much fungus

Oranges, spinach, Tomatoes = Too acidic

Salt = Results in potassium deficiency and water retention

Sugar = the killer! It disturbs blood glucose levels, causing disturbed appetite and energy levels.

Congratulations on reading this book and I hope you *will* change your eating habits and make it a part of your Life!

None of this is difficult to do in PRACTICAL terms, But psychologically? That's a different matter entirely. First you need to decide whether your eating habit is in charge - or YOU are...

If you have enjoyed reading my book can you please review it?

There is a Colouring Journal and Food Diary to help you change. It is available from Amazon.com books which is part of this series.

I have two Face Book pages with regards to Health:

Diets by Sue

Use and 'like' to get some extra tips and ideas.

Sue Feldman (NUT)

NOTES to remember:

www.ingramcontent.com/pod-product-compliance
Lightning Source LLC
Chambersburg PA
CBHW040322010626
45792CB00024B/2095